I0420659

The Devil Made Me Eat That!

By

C. M. Fleming

THE DEVIL MADE ME EAT THAT! Copyright 2015 by C. M. Fleming.

Cover photograph by Will Clark

Manufactured in the United States of America. All rights reserved.
No part of this book may be reproduced in any form or by any electronic
or mechanical means, including information storage and retrieval systems,
without permission in writing from the author, except by a reviewer, who
may quote brief passages in a review.

ISBN-13: 978-1517328832

ALSO BY C.M. FLEMING

Finder's Magic

Halley's Hope

The Devil Made Me Eat That!

By

C. M. Fleming

Acknowledgements, warnings, and disclaimers:

I am not a doctor, nutritionist, or physical trainer. Nor do I have a degree in theology, but I am a Christian, and a student of the Bible. I am a voracious reader on many subjects. My strongest qualification is that I have up close and personal experience with food addiction, and recovery. Like any addict, I am not cured, but struggle every day to resist the cravings.

Weight loss is big business. The diet industry doesn't' want you to find a permanent solution to your weight problem. If we were all to do so, these programs would go broke. This should raise a forest of red flags for anyone who is tempted to try the latest, greatest weight-loss gimmick.

The principles in this book are NOT intended as a solution for Bulimia, Anorexia, or other deep-seated emotional problems. If you suspect any of these conditions,

SEEK PROFESSIONAL MEDICAL HELP.

Before changing your eating habits, caloric intake, or exercise regimen – CHECK WITH YOUR DOCTOR. What I offer is a Biblically based, common sense approach to healthy eating and weight control, with a generous helping of humor.

This did not happen overnight. I didn't wake up one morning to discover that I was suddenly obese. In the same token, I didn't wake up one morning and see a slender senior staring back from the mirror. Both processes took time.

Chapter 1
In The Beginning (Where it All Started)

It's all because of the acceptable sin.

"Nonsense," you say. Everyone knows there is no such thing. But, you're curious. Am I right?

Well, you are correct. There is no such thing as an acceptable sin. There is something we as Christians not only accept, but encourage. It is the sin of gluttony. Don't believe me? Then you've never attended a good old-fashioned church "Potluck Dinner." We accept and encourage the act, but condemn the sinner.

"Okay," you say. "But a potluck dinner is not a sin – it's *fellowship*."

He who keeps the law is a discerning son, but a
companion of gluttons disgraces his father. Proverbs: 28:7

I am not saying that church members are gluttons, and to be fair, I can't blame it all on "fellowships." Everywhere we look there are enticements. Pick up a magazine. The cover touts "Lose 30 Pounds in Three Weeks!" or "Walk Off # Pounds by the Holidays," "New Medical Breakthrough: Melt Fat Away!" Inside there may be a two-page spread, detailing a diet, an exercise plan, or the latest over-the-counter pill, complete with before and after pictures of people for whom the plan, diet, or pill worked. (Can we say "Photo Shop"?) Compare that to the one hundred or so pages of tempting recipes, coupons, and restaurant ads.

Turn on your television and watch stick-thin actors consuming pizzas, burgers, French fries, burritos, fried chicken, etc. The list goes on and on. These commercials are often followed by advertisements for Weight Watchers, Jennie Craig, Nutrisystem, and countless others. Or they tell you to buy the newest exercise equipment. (Did you know they make great clothing racks? And what is that little timer/counter thing? Earned drying time?)

And while Weight Watchers, Jenny Craig and Nutrisystem work for a season, they are temporary fixes. Unless you make permanent behavior changes, you will go back to your old eating habits and gain back all the weight, and probably more.

When all that fails – and it will – you could always have liposuction, or have your stomach stapled, banded, or bypassed. But these so-called cures all have one huge risk factor in common – they could kill you! And none of them address the real issue. You have a food addiction. And guess what? It shows.

Thus, by their fruits ye will know them. Matthew 7:20

Before you condemn me for taking the above passage of scripture out of context, consider to whom Jesus was referring – false teachers. Would you consider someone who tells you "Buy my food, pill, or program, and you will lose weight, and your problems will be solved forever," a false teacher? I do.

Weight Watchers does have a long-term plan, and it has worked for thousands of people. There are also a lot of people who have been successful with them for a season, and then returned to their old habits – this author being among them.

As a matter of fact, I've tried just about every diet plan known to the human race. None of them permanently addressed my problem, because they left God out of the solution.

Many obese people blame God. God did not make you fat. God made you in His image.

Your dysfunctional family did not make you fat. You did not "think" yourself fat, therefore, you cannot think yourself thin. The problem does have to do with the way you think, but we will deal with that in a later chapter.

I do not have deep-seated emotional problems or use food as a crutch. I don't have a health condition such as low thyroid, hypo-, or hyperglycemia. My parents did not force me to clean my plate when I was a child. I was not deprived of love, nor was I abused. I have a loving, supportive husband, and great kids. I admit to using food for comfort in times of stress, but I also turn to food in celebration. For me, the real problem is what I call "food lust." I *LOVE* food – all kinds of food, but especially the high-calorie kind. And I'm not crazy about exercise.

I believe that many of you reading this are like me.

I'm not discounting emotional eating disorders like anorexia, and bulimia. These are serious health concerns that **require serious professional help**. Food addictions, whether eating too much, purging afterwards, or starving yourself, can kill you.

I find it ironic that the first sin involved disobedience concerning food. Consider this Biblical warning of deadly food.

The Lord took the man and put him in the Garden of Eden to work it

and take care of it. And the Lord God commanded the man,

"You are free to eat from any tree in the garden, but you must

not eat from the tree of the knowledge of good and evil,

for <u>when you eat of it, you will surely die</u>."

(Emphasis is mine) Genesis 2:15 – 17

Hmm, did He say "when," not "if?" God knows us so well.

Enter the tempter.

Now the serpent was more crafty than any of the wild animals the Lord God had made. He said to the woman, "Did God really say, 'You must not eat from any tree in the garden."? Genesis 3:1

Poor Eve, she got the warning second-hand, and added a little extra caution of her own. Or perhaps Adam, wanting to impress upon her the danger, told her they must not even touch that particular fruit.

Allow me a little sanctified imagination, if you will. We don't know what the fruit actually was, or what it looked like. (I'm thinking it might have looked and smelled a lot like a giant Krispy Kreme Donut.) Can't you just imagine that serpent coiling around it? *He* is touching it, his tongue flicking out, drawing in the fragrance of that forbidden delicacy. Can you hear his mocking tone? He taunts Eve, telling her it won't kill her, but will make her like God. Eve's mouth begins to water. Her eyes glaze over. She is drawn to it. Her hand has a will of its own. She reaches out and touches the fruit. Horrified, she jerks her hand away. Holding her breath, she waits for death – but she doesn't drop dead!

What was it the serpent said? *It would make them like God.* What if he's right? After all, he was right about it not killing her when she touched it.

The woman and man succumbed to temptation and ate the fruit. Did they die? Yes – not instantly, but the minute they disobeyed God, their bodies began to die, cell by cell.

Just as we have an inborn sin nature, we also have the desire to improve ourselves. We want to be more like God. And today, many, many centuries after Adam and Eve disobeyed God, we are still killing ourselves with food.

Chapter Two
Where Do We Go From Here?

Must we wander in the diet desert for forty years, living on mysterious manna that falls from the sky, and quails delivered by ravens? Or can we cross over into a land of milk and honey?

I vote for the latter. Actually, make mine cheesecake, please.

This is a book about weight loss! How can I even mention "CHEESECAKE?"

I realize it's very early in the book to reveal the *secret*, but here it is... Are you ready for the truth?

> *Do not withhold your mercy from me, O Lord; may your love and your truth always protect me. Psalm 40:11*

(Weight-loss Secret: Part I)

It's not about the type of food you eat.

That's right. Do you realize that guinea pigs get fat eating lettuce? And they don't even smother it with high-calorie dressings. (Which is what really distinguishes humans from lower life forms – Salad dressing.)

(Weight-loss Secret: Part II)

It's the volume of food you consume.

Guinea pigs are little guys, but they have to eat a lot of lettuce to get fat.

It's the volume combined with activity.

Pair eating too much food with an inactive lifestyle, and voila! Weight gain. You can put an exercise wheel in a guinea pig's cage, but you can't make him work out.

We are a generation of guinea pigs stuffing our chubby cheeks with tons of salad and diet soda. An hour later we are starving so we look for a snack. We justify this because *we only had a salad for lunch.* Whether it's a bag of chips, a doughnut, or a candy bar, to be on the safe side, we'll wash our snack down with another diet soda.

Put in a different way, weight gain or loss is directly related to the amount of food we eat and the amount of energy we expend. If we ingest more food or calories than we burn, we will gain weight. And conversely, if we burn more calories than we consume, we will lose weight.

It truly IS that simple. *And* that hard.

(Secret Part IV which is really Secret Part I)

You have to decide to do it.

That's right, secrets part I, II, and III don't mean a thing if you don't set your mind to do this thing. No matter what, just *DO IT*. There has to be a head change before there can be a body change.

Remember the Bible verse about how we are wonderfully made? Keep in mind that we were not cut out with a giant cookie cutter in heaven. We are each the same, but yet marvelously different. Therefore, there is no *one* formula that fits all.

Here is where it gets a little less "simple." No two people have exactly the same metabolic rate. Many variables factor into this; body build, bone structure, age, and gender. If you are like me, and have a very efficient or slow metabolism, you are able to maintain your body weight on fewer calories than others. Look on the bright side. If there were a famine, we would most likely survive.

It will take some trials and errors to learn how many calories your body requires to lose, gain, or maintain. I will tell you what worked for me, but I'm not going to give you diet menus, specific caloric guidelines or the number of points you may eat. The internet is a wonderful tool. There are many websites that tell you how many calories you need on a daily basis. The Mayo Clinic is a respected medical organization. They offer a calorie calculator at, http://www.mayoclinic.com/health/coloric-calculator/NUoo509. Or you can type "weight loss" into your search engine and start surfing. Unfortunately, your email inbox will be flooded with spam advertisements on weight loss products and programs. See a listing of other resources at the end of this book.

But even the respected Mayo Clinic can only give general guidelines. This site says that at my current age, weight, and activity level, I would maintain at 1750 calories a day. I know from past experience that this is too many calories for me. So I plugged in my desired weight, with NO activity. The result, 1500 calories a day. *I wish!*

It is possible that my extremely low metabolism rate is a direct result of years of yoyo dieting. I had to figure out a specific formula that worked for me.

In the beginning, err on the side of moderation. Start with a sensible amount. Use the Mayo Clinic site, or another calorie calculator. Combine this with some healthy physical activity. Don't be discouraged if you don't lose immediately. Keep in mind that you didn't wake up one morning as an obese person. If after a week of honestly, and accurately keeping track of how much food you've consumed, you have not lost any weight, reduce your intake slightly, or increase your activity. Even if you haven't lost weight yet, you are forming some healthy habits that will continue to help you throughout life.

On the other hand, don't get overconfident if you lose a lot of weight in the very beginning. Understand that it's probably water-weight, and the solid-packed-in-there fat will hang on for dear life. When the weight loss slows, stay with it.

Don't get crazy. The goal is to get healthy. If you starve yourself, you will lose weight temporarily, but you can't continue to eat that way. You will be tempted to binge, starting a vicious and dangerous circle.

Chapter Three
The Scales, Friend or Foe

It is easy to allow the scales to become too important. Remember that a set of scales is a tool, nothing more. Don't be obsessed with the number, and don't be controlled by the instrument but *do* use it as a measure.

You shall have no other gods before me. Exodus 20:3 (NIV)

One of my *thin* friends says, "I refuse to let the scales rule my life." I understand her concern with a number obsession, but for me that statement makes about as much sense as saying "I refuse to let the speedometer rule my driving." Try saying that to the traffic cop who asks you, "Do you know how fast you were driving?"

I need tools to help me stay on the right path, whether it is driving within the speed limit, or keeping my weight under control.

I struggle as I write this. The more I think about food, the more food I want to eat – not just eat, but *overeat.*

In the winter, a small group of my writer friends and I go to the beach for a week long writing retreat. At least, that's what we call it. We are all excellent cooks, and we all have a food addiction, (although the others may take umbrage with that statement.) It's akin to sending a group of alcoholics to a winery for a week. Each person is responsible for one evening meal. We plan, we schedule, and we salivate over menus. And unlike recovering alcoholics, we can't abstain from food, completely. We *have* to eat.

Invariably, one or more of us are on a "diet." The rest of the group lends support by cooking low calorie, low fat dishes, and trying to figure out which wine goes best with cottage cheese.

We do not bring bathroom scales with us, and there are none in our cottages. When I asked why that is, I got a couple of different answers. One doesn't own a set of scales. Another offered that I was free to bring scales if they fit in my suitcase. Space is limited, so I've chosen not to include that item. For me, there may be a deeper reason.

During a recent retreat, we passed a giant pay-to-weigh machine at a grocery store, and one friend asked if I wanted to check my weight. I nearly shouted my answer. "No!"

(I noticed that no one else hopped on the scales, either.)

Why? Let me count my reasons: 1. I was fully clothed. 2. It was right after lunch at our favorite seafood restaurant 3. I'd have to face reality, and… 4. EVERYONE else would know how much I weigh.

Logically, I know my weight loss or gain is obvious. I can camouflage to a degree, but it still shows. I don't eat in secret (now), so everyone in the group knew how much I had consumed. Another sin rears its ugly head – pride.

> *When pride comes, then comes disgrace, but*
> *with humility comes wisdom. Proverbs 11:2*

The thesaurus lists arrogance, conceit, and egotism, among others, as alternate words for pride. The antonym of pride is humility. I am proud of my accomplishment of losing weight, and if I had gained weight, I would have had to admit failure.

Don't judge me too harshly. Does your drivers' license list your true weight? Go ahead and keep your ugly little secret, or try to. Just remember – it all shows *in the end*. (Pun intended.)

So when is the best time to weigh? Is it better to weigh only once a month, once a week, or every day? The simple answer is, "whatever works best for you." For me, it is daily, right after I get up and while still wearing my lightweight pajamas.

In order to see the most accurate results of gaining, or losing weight, you should weigh at the same time of day, wearing the same clothing, or lack of.

In the beginning, your weight may fluctuate quite a bit. The thought behind once-a-week, or monthly weighing, is that you will become discouraged when you show a gain one day, and give up. If you go into this with the knowledge that this is not only a possibility, but a probability, you can keep working toward your goal.

The number on the scales motivates me. If the number is lower, (happy dance) I'm encouraged to keep working. If the number is higher, (no happy dance) I'm even more determined to stay the course until the number goes down.

A set of scales is not a god to bow down to, but your friend. A friend will tell you the truth, even if it hurts.

Chapter Four
The Seven Deadly Sins
Vs.
The Ten Commandments

God does not qualify sin as man does. "The Seven Deadly Sins" is a list of the worst sins according to mankind.

The consequences of committing the seven deadly sins seem to be more relevant to physical health, i.e. "deadly," while the Ten Commandments are geared toward spiritual health.

Do you see how the seven deadly sins could relate to food addiction, or weight control?

Let's break them down.

1. Lust: overwhelming desire. I would say that I lust for certain foods – many foods.

2. Gluttony: is self-explanatory, eating more food than your body needs.

3. Greed: have you ever hidden a favorite snack from the rest of the family?

4. Sloth: an old fashioned word that means plain ol' laziness. Nuff said.

5. Wrath: do you feel angry if someone finds your stash and eats it all? Those greedy children! They're the reason you hid it in the first place.

6. Envy: oh to be able to eat anything you want and stay thin like _____. Fill in the blank.

7. Pride: too many years I denied that I had a food addiction problem and wouldn't accept help. I ate in secret, wore baggy, fat-hiding clothing, and put on a fake happy face. Now that my addiction is under control, I must guard against a "holier-than-thou" attitude. I didn't do it on my own. God gets all the credit for changing my mind, and my body.

Now consider the Ten Commandments.

1. You shall have no other gods before me.
Don't let food or your weight become the most important thing in your life.

2. You shall not make for yourself an idol…
Do you idolize a celebrity for his or her appearance? Or do you bow before the false god of the scales?

3. You shall not misuse the name of the Lord your God…
Maybe not this one.

4. Remember the Sabbath day by keeping it holy.
Does your mind wander during a church service to which restaurant you will go to if the preacher will *ever* stop talking? Never mind that you are causing someone to have to work on the Sabbath.

5. Honor your father and mother.
Did your parents have a weight problem? If so, honor them by breaking the pattern.

6. You shall not murder.
Are you killing yourself with food?

7. You shall not commit adultery.

Okay, maybe not this one either, unless your illicit love of food is more important than family.

8. You shall not steal.

Our country wastes enough food to feed all the starving children in the world. Is that not akin to stealing? Also refer to commandment number 6.

9. You shall not give false testimony against your neighbor.

Hmmm, would lying about your weight on your driver's license count?

> 10. You shall not covet your neighbor's wife, house, servants, or
> livestock.

(Or his bountiful table.)

Moses received the Ten Commandments, "inscribed by the finger of God." I'd say that many of them relate to food addiction. Are you guilty of any of these? I am.

James, the brother of Jesus said,

> *For whoever keeps the whole law and yet stumbles at just one*
> *point is guilty of breaking all of it. James 2:10 NIV*

So what's a hopeless food addict to do? Are we destined to spend eternity in diet hell? Did you not read chapter two? Re-read it, and then proceed directly to chapter five. Do not pass "go." Do not collect 2,000 calories. I mean $200.

Chapter Five
Food...
This Ain't No Thinkin' Thang

This ain't no thinkin' thing, right brain, left brain
It goes a little deeper than that
It's a chemical, physical, emotional devotion
Passion that we can't hold back
There's nothin` that we need to analyze
There ain't no rhyme or reason why
'Cause this ain't, this ain't no thinkin` thing
(Song written by: Tim Nichols & Mark Sanders. Recorded by:
Trace Atkins)

That kind of thinking, or non-thinking, is what got us here in the first place, whether it's a bad relationship with food, or with a person. Stop living in the land of too much milk and honey. The land is full of giants, and they are us.

The children of Israel needed written instructions for life. Likewise, we need written guidelines for a proper relationship with God, and with food. We need the equivalent of a mezuzah.

A mezuzah is a daily reminder — and a public declaration — of Jewish identity and faith. The mezuzah is affixed to the doorframe in Jewish homes to fulfill the *mitzvah* (Biblical commandment) to inscribe the words of the Shema "on the doorposts of your house" (Deuteronomy 6:9).

On certain things I am a slow learner. People learn by reading, hearing, *and* practicing. Some people only need one method, but I need all three.

You could say that I am calorically dyslexic. I've tried to keep track of calories in my head, but that simply doesn't work for me. Also, I have a little-known condition called Food Consumption Amnesia. We will call it FCA. The only known treatment for FCA is to keep a food journal, a mezuzah, if you will. (You will find a sample journal at the end of this book. Feel free to copy it and use it.) For all you techie geeks, there are some wonderful apps available for your computer or iPhone. One of my skinny friends uses an app called "Lose It." She looks fabulous. She didn't have a lot to lose, but that last twenty or so pounds can be the toughest. The app helps you keep track of the food you eat, and how many calories you burn while exercising. There are comparable sites on the internet, as well.

The key is honesty. If you eat a spoonful of peanut butter while making your children, or in my case, grandchildren, a PB&J sandwich – write it down. Those calories count, too.

Sorry Trace, it *is* a thinkin' thang.

Chapter Six
Get Off Your Gluteus Maximus!

Wasn't he a Roman Emperor?

In chapter two, I stated that you should include a certain level of exercise to burn calories and lose weight. My chosen profession is in direct conflict with that concept. I am a writer, which means that I sit in front of a computer much of the time. So what is the solution? It is as plain as the spare tire around my middle – planned exercise. Set a time for activity, and just DO IT. It doesn't have to be jogging, weight lifting, or ab crunches. Simply stated, start moving. Do that "E" thing (exercise) that we hate almost as much as we hate the "D" word (diet).

That being said, I cannot overemphasize how important it is to check with your physician before starting any exercise program.

A writer-friend of mine suggests sitting on a balance, or exercise ball while writing. I'm not that coordinated. A gym membership is worth my weight in gold. While working to lose weight, I worked out five days a week. Now, in maintenance I go to the gym as often as my schedule permits. Sometimes it is only once a week. I almost wrote "try to go." A quote from Yoda, of Star Wars fame, is apropos here. "There is no try. Try *not*. Do."

Don't use your age as an excuse for not exercising. Did you read the first page where I revealed that I am over 69 years old? In addition to that fact, I have osteoarthritis in my knees, which makes certain activities very painful. In the beginning, my husband and I invested in the services of a personal trainer who specializes in older clients. Her fee was reasonable, and she knew what she was doing. As I gained strength, and lost weight, movement became easier. Soon we were flying solo. We are living geriatric proof that you can lose weight at any age.

Many insurance plans, especially those for the "senior" crowd, will pay for gym membership. It's called "Silver Sneakers." Insurance companies are finally realizing that it's more cost-effective to keep you healthy than to fix a problem later. A recent study has revealed that exercise, or simple movement of any kind helps ward off Alzheimer's disease. What a plus!

But you don't absolutely *have* to exercise in a gym. Many city parks have wonderful paved walking or jogging trails. Check out a local high school track after hours. Most tracks are a quarter of a mile, making it easy to keep track of the distance you walk. It is a good idea to have a walking partner. There is safety in numbers, and a partner will hold you accountable. You have the added responsibility of encouraging your partner, as well.

Though one may be overpowered, two can defend themselves.
A cord of three strands is not quickly broken. Ecclesiastes 4:12

Walking may not be your exercise of choice. Or perhaps you don't have time to *go* somewhere to exercise because you have to clean your house. Put on some lively music and vacuum your floors to a rockin' beat. Find an "oldies" radio station and find out how much fun it can be to dance in the kitchen. Stir that sauce (low calorie, of course) to "Twistin' the Night Away." I love to play Salsa music while cooking Mexican Food. Who can resist moving to a Latin beat?

If you want some inexpensive weights, cans of food from your pantry are the perfect solution. And you would be surprised to learn how much a gallon of liquid weighs.

If you own, or have access to a swimming pool, that is an excellent way to work off pounds. Not a very good swimmer? Neither am I. Try walking quickly back and forth across the shallow end, or hold onto the side of the pool and kick your legs vigorously. Exercising in water has low impact on bad knees, and the water gives resistance, helping to burn calories.

Don't be shocked, or upset to see a higher number on the scales the day after an intense workout. My husband likes to remind me that muscle is heavier than fat. I like to counter with, "A *pound* of muscle weighs the same as a *pound* of fat."

He is right, but don't tell him I said so. Not only is muscle heavier than fat, *sore muscles* hold fluid, making them temporarily even heavier.

Keep in mind that muscle burns more calories than fat. Therefore, while building muscle improves your appearance, an added benefit is a boost in your metabolism. Exercise gives a lazy metabolism a kick-start, too. A win, win situation!

Chapter Seven
Off to See the Wizard

Who wouldn't welcome a little magical help with a difficult problem?

I'm reminded of the movie, "The Wizard of Oz." Dorothy and friends had some major personal problems that needed super-natural help, so they headed down the Yellow Brick Road through many dangers and snares until they finally reached The Emerald City, the home of the Great and Powerful Oz.

At last their problems would be solved. But it turned out that it wasn't so easy to get an audience with the wizard. First, each had to undergo a complete makeover, hair, nails, rust removal, etc.

Ladies, can you identify with that? If we have a great hairdo, perfect makeup, and an immaculate manicure, maybe no one will notice our other physical faults.

Don't laugh men. You are no different. Do you think if you color your gray hair no one will notice that pot-belly? Perhaps a stylish beard will camouflage a double chin. Think again. You will still be a guy with a pot-belly, but now with brown hair. The beard will *cover* both chins, but not *hide* them.

When Dorothy, the Cowardly Lion, Scarecrow, and Tin Man were deemed presentable, they were ushered into the chamber of the great man, himself! Timidly, with much trembling, one by one they made their requests. And what did the great and powerful Oz do? He told them he would happily grant each wish, but with one minor string attached. First, they had to kill the Wicked Witch!

How in the world could mere mortals accomplish such an impossible task? Even though they didn't have a clue, the brave little quartet set out to give it their best shot. You know the rest of the story. They succeeded, but the Wizard didn't really have any supernatural powers to grant their wishes.

You might say, but *that's* fiction, and it is. You may be surprised to learn that we have some modern-day wizards in our midst. They appear on television. Dr. Oz (notice the similarity in names) often shares weight loss tips. Recently he praised the miraculous properties of safflower oil. This oil will supposedly melt away belly fat. There is an expensive product you can buy and drink daily. The concept is that you don't have to change your diet or amount of exercise.

If you increase calories and don't increase activity, YOU WILL GAIN WEIGHT. I know this because I tried adding safflower oil to my diet and gained weight right away. Will I never learn?

Another popular TV personality is Dr. Phil. He is well known for his folksy sayings, "Get real," and "How's that workin' for ya?" He says that 95% of people on a diet gain weight. And the next thing we know he is hawking a new book "The Seventeen Day Diet" and another one especially for women entitled "P.I.N.K.," like an old-time medicine man.

Quick! I gotta get me some of that snake oil!

Both of these books, though not written by Dr. Phil, are published and sold online by his son. *Get real, Doc! If we buy these books, we probably won't lose weight, but we'll make your family richer.*

How's that workin' for ya? Quite well if you're the good doctor!

Pay no attention to those men behind the (television) screen.

I hate and abhor falsehood but I love your law. Psalm 119: 163 (NIV)

Don't get me wrong, I enjoy watching both of their shows. I also like to read a good book, especially fiction.

It may be cliché, but if it sounds too good to be true, it probably is.

Dear friends do not believe every spirit, but test the spirits to see whether they are from God, because many false prophets have gone out into the world. I John 4:1 (NIV)

This brings me to another popular, albeit extreme, method of weight loss – gastric bypass surgery. Please, please do not go this route. It drastically changes your body and digestive system. If you live through the surgery, you will probably lose a lot of weight in a short time. But people have been known to gain all the weight back, even though their stomach is the size of a walnut.

Don't you know that you yourselves are God's temple and that God lives in you? If anyone destroys God's temple, God will destroy him; for God's temple is sacred, and you are that temple, I Cor. 3:16-17 (NIV)

I personally know a morbidly obese man who chose to have the bariatric surgery. During surgery, he had a stroke and his heart actually stopped beating. The doctors were able to revive him, but they couldn't reverse today the damage done by the stroke. Now, many years later, he is an invalid, and still morbidly obese.

A couple of years ago, another acquaintance had the less drastic lap-band surgery. It was to be an out-patient procedure, but again there were complications and he had to stay in the hospital. As far as I know, he had no other problems and was released a few days later. I don't know how many pounds he has lost, but it's been two years, and his weight loss doesn't appear to be significant.

A weight problem doesn't start in your stomach. It starts in your head. In an earlier chapter I said "you can't think yourself thin." I promised to address that in a later chapter. While it is true that thinking, alone, will not make the weight come off, changing the way you think about food can go a long way toward helping your meet your weight goal, as long as you follow that change with the positive action.

Chapter Eight
Babylonian Captivity

One of my all-time favorite Bible heroes is Daniel. The book of Daniel opens at the time when King Jehoiakim, Daniel's father, was killed by Nebuchadnezzar, king of Babylon. The holy temple was looted and priceless religious articles were stolen and placed in the treasure house of a pagan god. These religious articles were not the most valuable things taken by the enemy. Jehoiakim's sons, Daniel and other princes of Judah were kidnapped to become slaves in the palace of the conquering king.

Try to imagine what these young boys experienced. Pampered princes of Judah accustomed to a life of wealth and privilege probably witnessed the murder of their father. Then they were forced to walk to a foreign land some nine hundred – NINE HUNDRED – miles away – to Babylon – Sin City. That's equivalent to walking from Tucson to Oklahoma City – in chains! This had to be the worst nightmare for a good Jewish boy, let alone a prince. But it gets worse.

The King James translation says,

And the king spake unto Ashpenas the master of his eunuchs,
that he should bring certain of the children of Israel
and of the king's seed, and of the princes; Daniel 1: 3 KJ

Does this mean that the young princes were made into eunuchs? Many scholars believe this to be the true. Castration was typically carried out on young males without their consent in order that they might perform a specific social functions; this was common in many societies. Was the King's reason for this so that the princes wouldn't father children who might later bring revenge on his kingdom, or was it yet another cruelty of conquest? I don't have the answer to that.

The passage goes on to detail how the young men were chosen.

Children in whom was no blemish, but well favoured, and skillful in all wisdom, and cunning in knowledge, and understanding science. And such as had ability in them to stand in the king's palace, and whom they might teach the learning and the tongue of the Chaldeans.
Daniel 1:4 KJ

So much for how far good looks and brains will take you!

But then the king ordered that the adolescents be fed the same rich meat and fine wine that was served at his table. No doubt this fare included foods that were strictly forbidden for Jews to eat. It goes even deeper than that.

In certain Eastern cultures sharing food, or a meal, is tantamount to a covenant. The Jews were taught from birth that they were God's chosen people, set apart. In other words, they were to remain separate from the pagan world.

Before you remind me that Jesus ate with sinners, I'd like to point out that these boys lived hundreds of years before Jesus. They were subject to the Old Testament covenant of "The Law." Jesus' life, death and resurrection changed the covenant.

Considering all that happened to these princes, wouldn't eating rich foods provided by the enemy be an *acceptable sin*? Daniel and his companions didn't think so. They chose to remain faithful to their heritage.

Four young men are mentioned by name, Daniel, Hananiah, Mishael, and Azariah. How I admire the integrity of these boys. (This is especially incomprehensible if you've ever tried to fill up teenaged boys.)

Nebuchadnezzar was probably the greatest ruler of the Neo-Babylonian period and one of the most competent monarchs of ancient times. His plan was to completely indoctrinate these Hebrew boys into the Babylonian culture. He knew how to conquer by might, and by mind control. He would break down their resolve with brutality and then with kindness.

In her study of Daniel, well-known Christian teacher and author, Beth Moore says, "Nothing is more dangerous than friendly captivity."

Even their Hebrew names, which all referenced the one true God, were changed to names associated with pagan gods. I feel certain the purpose in this was to bring about total immersion into Babylonian culture, mind, body, and soul.

Daniel resolved not to defile himself by eating forbidden, unhealthy food. Remember that the boys were chosen because they were blessed with above average intelligence. Daniel's actions prove that he *was* smart. Rather than blatantly defy the king's orders, He went directly to the man in charge over their care, Ashpenaz, with a request that the four be allowed to eat only fruit, grains and vegetables. The following includes the official's response.

Now God had caused the official to show favor and sympathy to Daniel,

but the official told Daniel, "I am afraid of my lord the king, who has assigned your food and drink. Why should he see you looking worse than the

other young men your age? The king would then have my head because of you."

Daniel 1;9-10 (NIV)

Daniel asked for a trial period of ten days to prove that they would remain healthy, and the official agreed.

I am not advocating that you go on a "Daniel diet." Daniel's purpose had nothing to do with weight loss. It had to do with yielding to sin or living a virtuous life. The scripture says…

At the end of ten days they looked healthier and better nourished than any of the young men who ate the royal food. Daniel 1:15

I can picture these impressionable boys, used to wealth and privilege, observing their opulent surroundings. They knew, first hand, the importance of appearances. At the king's directive, they were probably clothed in the best Babylonian couture. I know they were slaves, but they were "special" slaves. Perhaps they were given some rad haircuts. Maybe they cruised around Babylon in the newest model of chariot. (Okay, I totally made all this up. Have I mentioned that I have a vivid imagination?)

My point with all this, and I do have a point, is that these four young men never gave in to the sin of disobedience concerning forbidden foods, gluttony, or the worship of pagan gods. God gave them strength to resist almost incomprehensible temptations. We are captive in a modern-day Babylon. There are temptations on every side. The family unit has all but fallen apart. There are children with no male role model because the father is either too busy making a living, or is not present in their lives at all. Children are not taught what food is good and healthy. It is easier for hard-working, busy parents, or caregivers to drive through a fast food restaurant and grab a sack of greasy burgers and fries – oh, and super-size that, please. Add a sugary drink and call it a meal.

If the God of Daniel could give these young boys wisdom and the strength of character to remain faithful under such dire circumstances, He can do the same for you and me as we fight the sin of gluttony. Sin is sin, is sin, is sin, but God is the same yesterday, today, and forever.

No temptation has seized you except what is common to man. And God is

faithful; he will not let you be tempted beyond what you can bear. But when you

are tempted, he will also provide a way out so that you can stand up under it.

I Cor. 10:13 (NIV)

As believers we have a freedom.

"Everything is permissible" – but not everything is beneficial.

"Everything is permissible" – but not everything is constructive.

I Cor 10:23

The bottom line is that we are free to choose, but we need to consider the consequences of our actions. Gluttony is a sin that has immediate and long lasting consequences. Let God's word guide your decisions, even when choosing what and how much to eat.

Chapter Nine
Celebrating With Food
(The Prodigal Son & Others)

Have I so completely weighed you down with guilt that you can never enjoy food again? That is not my intention. There are numerous accounts in the Bible of times when God's people celebrated with food. One such is the story of "The Prodigal Son," a parable told by Jesus. It begins in Luke 15:12

No doubt you've heard this story, but I'll recount it here. First you need to know a little about the customs of the time. At a man's death, most of his worldly possessions were left to the eldest son. Second and consequent sons received a smaller portion. Daughters received nothing. They were supposed to marry and be supported by a husband. Fathers did provide a dowry for daughters, but it went straight to a husband, not the daughter herself.

The focus of the story of the Prodigal Son is the younger son. Apparently he saw no future in his position as the minor son. He went to his father and asked for all of his inheritance paid in advance.

I find it pretty amazing that the father complied with this request. Minor son; let's call him "Bubba." So Bubba hits the road, not the Yellow Brick Road, but he is definitely in search of an Emerald City. He is dazzled by the sights, sounds, and smells of city living. There are temptations on every corner – literally. Bubba is everybody's friend, buying drinks, food, and "entertainment" – that is until his money runs out. Do you get the idea that Bubba ain't the brightest candle on the Menorah?

Poor Bubba, his pockets are empty and his "friends" are gone. Doors slam in his face, people turn their backs on him when he approaches. He can't find a job because he has no skills, and he can't go home because he burned that bridge. What's a po' boy to do?

Just outside of town lives a pig farmer, obviously not Jewish, but Bubba is desperate. He swallows his pride and gets a job feeding the swine. Even pig slop begins to look good, so Bubba eats some. Imagine the pigs' surprise at the appearance of a Jewish dinner guest.

Finally, Bubba comes to his senses, what little he has. He remembers that even the workers on his father's farm eat far better than this. It won't be easy, but he will humble himself, go home, and beg his father's forgiveness and ask to work for him.

I am going resist preaching to you here, but look for it sooner or later.

As Bubba nears his father's farm, Daddy sees him coming. Daddy is overjoyed. He hikes up his robes and hoofs it down the road to meet his baby boy.

We don't know how long Bubba was gone, weeks, months or years, but whatever the length of time, the father hadn't known if his son was alive or dead. Now here he is, looking more dead than alive, and probably smelling worse. Daddy weeps with joy. He throws his arms around his son and kisses him.

Then Daddy pulls himself together and orders the servants to "kill the fatted calf." He tells them to put the best robe on Bubba, a ring on his finger, and sandals on his feet.

Number one son, Jr. has been home all this time, working on the family farm, like a good son. He is working in the fields when Bubba returns. Jr. comes in, hot tired and dirty to find a party going on. He asks one of the servants who explains everything. Jr. is so angry he refuses to go inside to the feast.

Daddy comes out and pleads with him to join them. Jr. lets Daddy have it.

But he answered his father, 'Look! All these years I've been slaving for
you and never disobeyed your orders. Yet you never gave me even a
young goat, so I could celebrate with my friends. But when this son of
yours who has squandered your property with prostitutes comes
home, you kill the fattened calf for him!" Luke 15:29-30 (NIV)

Notice how he calls his brother, "this son of yours."

Daddy answers:

'My son,' the father said, 'you are always with me, and everything I
have is yours.
But we had to celebrate and be glad, because this brother of yours
was dead

and is alive again; he was lost and is found.' Luke 15:31-32

The father brings it back to him by saying, "this brother of yours."

I've always sympathized with Jr. Now that I'm older and have children of my own, I can understand the father's feelings. Just because his son made foolish decisions didn't mean he loved him any less.

(Warning: Preaching ahead)

This is how our heavenly Father feels about us. He loves us unconditionally. And who among us had not made foolish decisions at one time or another? He is overjoyed when we return to Him and ask for His help. I believe we'll be greeted with a celebration feast in heaven.

The older son had always done the right thing, but when his brother returned he committed the double sins of pride and covetousness. He judged his brother and found him lacking. Like Jr., we are in no position to judge our brothers or sisters.

(End of preaching, for the time being.)

Another Biblical account of celebrating with food is found in the Old Testament book of Nehemiah.

Nehemiah, a servant to conquering king Artaxerxes (try saying that three times in a row) was given permission to return to Jerusalem, his homeland, to oversee the rebuilding of the city walls and the holy temple of God. Besides letting the house of God fall into total disrepair, the people had been living a sinful life, marrying pagans and practicing forbidden ceremonies.

In spite of much enemy opposition, Nehemiah was able to organize the people to reconstruct the walls and the temple. At the dedication Ezra, the scribe brought out the Book of the Law of Moses. They had an all day, old fashioned tent revival.

At the end of the day, the people wept in repentance. Read what happened:

> *Then Nehemiah the governor, Ezra the Priest and scribe, and the Levites*
> *who were instructing the people said to them all, "This day is sacred to the*
> *Lord your God. Do not mourn or weep." For all the people had been weeping as they listened to the words of the Law. Nehemiah said, "Go and enjoy choice food and sweet drinks, and send some to those who have nothing prepared. This day is sacred to our Lord. Do not grieve, for the joy of the Lord is your strength."*
> *Nehemiah 8:9-10*

So there we have the first recorded church pot-luck fellowship. They celebrated with "choice" food. My mouth is watering at the thought of creamy cheese topped with sweetened figs.

There are many other accounts of feasts for one holiday or another. Notice that the scripture doesn't say that they had a food orgy. Enjoying food is okay, as long as we don't take it as far as the act of gluttony.

Chapter Ten
The Great Pyramid
(Food Pyramid, that is.)

The currently accepted food chart is a divided plate, but I wanted an ancient symbol, so I asked myself, "What would Pharaoh do?" He would build a pyramid, of course, and fill it with all the food he would need in the afterlife.

(Insert illustration of food pyramid here)

There have been changes to the food pyramid over the years, and though there are other charts and graphs as I mentioned, the pyramid is still a reasonable guide of what you should eat each day based on governmental dietary guidelines. Remember that the pyramid is a general guide, not a rigid prescription. It shows what is considered a healthful diet for most people. It includes a variety of foods to get all the nutrients you need.

Jews were taught that certain food was forbidden. We saw the importance of observing these rules in the recount of Daniel. Some Jewish people still observe these rules; it is called "keeping kosher." The New Testament teaches that no foods are forbidden, (but gluttony is.) In the tenth chapter of Acts, Peter falls into a trance and has a vision of unclean animals being presented to him for food. He was told to kill and eat. His response was:

> *"Surely not, Lord" Peter replied. "I have never eaten anything impure or*

unclean." The voice spoke to him a second time, "Do not call anything

impure that God has made clean." Acts 10:14-15

With that in mind, let's start at the top of the pyramid and work down, kind of like eating dessert first. The tip of the pyramid represents the smallest amount of dietary requirements in the complete profile. Note that it includes fats, oils and sweets. Yes, fats and oils *are* a dietary *requirement,* but more on this at the end of the chapter. Sweets are less important because your digestive system turns other things into glucose, or sugar.

As we work our way down the pyramid – do you feel a little like Indiana Jones – the next level is dairy, meat, fish, poultry, dry beans, eggs, and nuts. This is the protein layer. Incidentally, these also contain fats, or oil, even dry beans, although there's a very small amount in beans. The recommended number of servings is two to three of dairy and two to three servings of any combination of the other foods in this category.

Drop down another level. What are those lovely colorful things, emeralds, rubies? Have we found the mummy's treasures? No it's just fruits and vegetables. Mummy says eat your veggies, three to five servings of a day. Two to four servings of fruit is advised.

Fresh is best, but isn't always readily available. Frozen is the next best alternative, and canned is better than skipping them.

Finally we have reached the ground floor, the base of the pyramid, and the foundation of our food requirements, bread, cereal, rice and pasta, or grain-based foods. In Jesus' day bread and grains were staples of their diet, and they still should be. Forget the Atkins Diet or the Carb Free Diet. Carbohydrates are NOT bad for you. Your body needs them. You should have six to eleven servings a day. That is more than any of the other food groups. Whole grains are the healthiest, and take the longest to digest, preventing hunger longer.

This is all well and good, but what is considered a serving? And here is where so many of us go wrong. Let me begin by telling you what a serving is *not*. A serving of cereal is not a full mixing bowl. A serving of dry cereal is one ounce, or one-half, to three-fourths of a cup. For bread, it is one slice and for cooked cereal it also one-half cup.

A serving of pasta is not a mountain of pasta piled on a twelve inch platter and smothered in sauce. It is one half cup. An average portion in a restaurant is typically about three servings.

A serving of vegetables is not a head of lettuce plus all the other good stuff. Not to mention salad dressing. Remember those portly little guinea pigs getting fat on lettuce? Leafy vegetables only require one cup. A serving of other vegetables, raw or cooked, is one-half cup. If you are going to overboard, this is the area to do it, as long as you don't smother them with bacon grease, butter, or sour cream.

Fruits are loaded with sugar – the natural kind, slower to be pumped into your bloodstream. While this is better than granulated or white sugar, keep in mind that they do become sugar in your bloodstream. One medium apple, banana, or orange is a serving. One half cup of chopped, cooked or canned fruit, without added processed sugar, is a reasonable amount. With juice, it is three-fourths of a cup, vegetable or fruit.

You get the idea. We've been super sizing our servings for too long. I'll stop telling what a serving isn't. Keep in mind that these are general guidelines. Depending on your body size, most people won't need the maximum number of servings of anything.

A serving of meat, poultry, or fish is two to three ounces. For a visual mental guide, that is about the size of your average computer mouse, or a deck of cards. One-half cup of cooked beans, one egg, or two tablespoons of peanut butter equal the same amount of protein as one ounce of lean meat.

We are nearly back to the top of the pyramid Mr. Jones, and we haven't encountered a single snake, or crocodile – although if you ate either, they would be listed in the protein level. I'm told that both taste a lot like chicken.

Here we are back at the summit where the category is fats, oils, and sweets. Serving sizes were not listed for these. The recommendation was to "use sparingly." So what fats should you eat, saturated, unsaturated, partially hydrogenated, omega-3s? In this era of the "fat-free" craze you will be happy to know that eating the good kind can actually tip the scales in your favor. Don't overindulge though, or the scales will tip in the wrong direction.

There are healthy oils and then there are the hit-man oils, lurking in your bloodstream waiting to bump you off when you least expect it. (Can you say heart attack, stroke, or cirrhosis?) The hit-man oils are man-made trans fats. They have been connected with increased bad (LDL) cholesterol and lower good (HDL) cholesterol. Unlike natural saturated fats like those in dairy products and meats, the man-made ones have been chemically altered through a process called "hydrogenation." in order to give them a longer shelf life.

The problem is, you may not even be aware that the bad oil is in a product because of tricky labeling laws that allow manufacturers to list zero grams of trans fat as long as a serving contains less than 0.5 grams. To avoid them, stay away from any product whose ingredients panel lists hydrogenated or partially hydrogenated oils.

Some of the good oils are olive, safflower, soy, cottonseed, peanut and nut oils. Be sure they are organic, as some crops, like cotton, is not regulated as a food crop, and is sprayed with strong pesticides and other chemicals. Remember, even good oils have calories. Sorry, do I sound like a broken cd? You still have to count them in your daily food intake. And since they are listed in the top of the food pyramid, I repeat, you should use them sparingly.

Fat has a serious image problem – a moment on the lips – a lifetime on the hips. Of course they make food taste better. It's no wonder Paula Deen's recipes are so delicious. "Put a little butter on it, y'all."

Our bodies need certain fats in order to utilize fat-soluble vitamins such as A, D, E, and K. If fat isn't available the vitamins can't be absorbed properly.

This isn't license to gorge on cinnamon rolls, doughnuts, and cheese fries. These items are the reason fat has such a bad image. Spread your fat-carb combinations sparingly throughout the day. Pairing fats and carbs in the same meal will keep our blood sugar stable and help prevent hunger longer. I'm referring to healthy fats, like that found in salmon, avocados, and nuts. A study in the journal *Diabetes Care* found that a diet rich in monounsaturated fats (such as almonds) may prevent the accumulation of abdominal fat.

I keep harping on calories. Here is a revelation for you. The new "fat-free" products are often higher in calories than the old-fashioned foods we used to think nothing of eating. Fact: CDC data shows that while Americans consumed a lower percentage of calories from fat in 2000 than they did in 1971, the total number of calories consumed by women per day increased by more than 300.

This is a direct result of manufacturers replacing the fat in foods with sugar. And that brings me to a whole other, but related topic; manufactured food. When manufacturers alter food, it is for their bottom line – profit – not your health.

Whole grains, certain non-processed foods are the most beneficial to your body. Fresh eggs from free-range chickens are amazingly delicious, and good for you. Dairy products are the exception. It's not a good idea to consume whole, raw milk if you don't know whether or not the cow has been tested for disease.

Have we gotten so smart that we've actually out-smarted ourselves? Don't trade whole organic food for manufactured food, and don't trade fat for sugar. Sugar contributes to belly fat.

Chapter Eleven
Love, Secrets, Lies and Half-truths

Ah food, how do I love thee? Let me count the ways; hot, cold, spicy, sweet, salty, sour, crunchy, and multiple combinations of the aforementioned. Not just food, though. There are other things I love, like pretty scarves, that hide double chins, over-sized blouses, stretchy pants, and wide-brimmed hats that balance the rest of me. But seriously, I love God, my family, and my country.

Perhaps "love" is the wrong word. We *enjoy* most of the things mentioned above. It is acceptable to love God, family, and country, but to say that we *love* those other things places too much importance on them.

In this great country, we have a government that looks out for our welfare with countless agencies to regulate everything from the food we eat to the air we breathe. And we all expect our government officials to tell us the truth. Don't we? Well, don't we?

Don't believe everything your government, news agencies, or advertisers tell you. Sometimes I feel like Jeremiah when he wrote:

"Friend deceives friend, and no one speaks the truth. They have taught their tongues to lie; they weary themselves with sinning. You live in the midst of deception; in their deceit they refuse to acknowledge me," declares the Lord. Jeremiah 9:5-6

So what are we to do?

Weigh everything with common sense. Don't fall for every new fad diet, weight-loss supplement, or exercise equipment. We are an enlightened generation. After all, we have Google! (I am tempted to insert a smiley face here.) Seriously, for every wild claim, you can usually find a repudiation if you will only take a few minutes to investigate. When you are tempted to rush to the phone with credit card in hand and dial that 800 number for a "Limited time only" special. Stop! Think! Google! You would be surprised how many times this simple action has saved me from spending money foolishly. Lest I come off sounding like a know-it-all – it took me a long time and a lot of wasted money to learn this. My hope is that you will learn from *my* mistakes.

Let's examine some of the common lies we've all heard, (or told ourselves.)

- **True or False:** You can't lose weight on your own.

False: You can't do it any other way. A support group can encourage, and inspire you, but eventually you have to be accountable for your own actions. No one else can do that for you.

- **True or False:** Obesity is in my genes.

It may be in your plus-size jeans, but it probably isn't in your DNA. More than likely, what your family did pass on to you is bad eating habits.

- **True or False:** You can't lose weight after age 40.

False: You require fewer calories later in life mainly because you are less active, and therefore burn fewer. Your body still works the same way. Calories in equals either fuel or stored fat. (I am way over 40.)

- **True or False:** The best way to lose weight is to eat only one meal a day.

This is one of the worst lies for several reasons. By the time you eat your "one" meal, you are starving and will probably eat much more than usual, justifying the amount because it's your only meal. Most people make it their evening meal and then go to bed, giving their body no opportunity to burn any of it off. Also, your digestive system is much more efficient at digesting large quantities of food than it is small amounts. Picture a conveyor belt taking a huge meal past a crew of tiny food factory workers, into your digestive tract. Quick, call in reinforcements! We've got a big job to do here! Every crumb of food is put to use, or stored on your hips, belly, and thighs. Then the reverse is true for a small meal. The tiny food worker supervisor sends all but one or two workers off to do other work. Picture the famous episode of "I Love Lucy," when Lucy and Ethyl go to work at the chocolate factory. Got that picture in your head? Some of the calories get rushed through and out the back door. Sorry to be graphic, but them's the facts.

- **True or False:** If you eat too few calories, your body goes into starvation mode and you will stop losing weight.

This is a half-truth. If you constantly starve yourself, your body does go into starvation, or self-preservation mode. If you continue to ignore your body's signals that you need fuel, you will lose weight, but you will be losing muscle rather than fat. The less lean muscle you have, the fewer calories your body will burn.

- **True or False:** You don't have to exercise to lose weight.

This is another half-truth. Exercise helps to burn off the food you've eaten. You can lose weight without exercising, but again, you are in danger of losing muscle mass.

- **True or False:** You can't eat bread, potatoes and desserts and still lose weight.

This is a complete lie. If you eliminate all starches from your diet, your body goes into a state of ketosis. This is a condition that causes the body to produce ketones, compounds believed by some to be harmful to your brain. Also a dangerous condition called ketoacidosis can develop in people with Type I Diabetes because it affects the insulin levels in your blood stream. (Information from mayoclinic.com.) It is best to consume lean protein with good carbohydrates, (like whole grains) because it allows your body to get the energy it needs without the added fat. Remember the food pyramid? Grain is the foundation. Whole grains give your digestive system the fiber it needs to keep food moving through, and fiber takes longer to digest. That gives you a "full" feeling for a longer time, making you less likely to seek a high calorie snack.

- **True or False:** Drinking diet sodas will make you skinny.

This one is not true either. Calorie free is better than drinking high-sugar drinks, but diet sodas may possibly cause you to gain more weight over time. It is not clear why, but your brain may anticipate calories when a drink tastes sugary, or fatty, so artificial sweeteners may actually cause cravings. Try kicking the diet Coke habit, or at least limit yourself to only one a day.

- **True or False:** Caffeinated drinks curb your appetite and boost your energy, causing you to lose weight more quickly.

Nope, sorry. Caffeine may suppress your appetite briefly, and give a slight increase in energy. It does not cause real, long-term weight loss. Caffeine also acts as a diuretic, can cause dehydration. It is a central nervous system stimulant which can affect our heart rate and blood pressure. It's a good idea to keep a check on the amount of caffeine you consume. This goes along with the information on diet drinks, many of which contain high concentrations of the stimulant.

- **True or False:** You should drink water to help with weight loss.

This is true. Water helps keep you hydrated and assists in flushing toxins from your body. A friend in the medical field told me that when fat breaks down, part of it turns to water. Drinking water helps rid your body of the fat squeezed from those plump little fat cells. It will even reduce the soreness of muscles after an especially vigorous workout. I'm sure you've heard the recommended amount of eight to ten 8 ounce glasses a day. This is good advice.

Chapter Twelve
Glycemic Index/Caloric Index/Carbs
(Foods you must never eat. Really?)

Warning: Technical jargon ahead, to show my smarts.

I am constantly seeing weight-loss ads that warn of "foods you should never eat." You don't have to have a PHD in nutrition to know that some foods are more fattening than others. I have stated that what you eat is not as important as how much you eat. I stand by that statement. If you choose to eat something with higher fat and calories, you must choose less of it.

So what's all this business about glycemic index? And what does it mean in terms of weight loss or gain? I did some investigating. As I understand it, the index ranks carbohydrates based on their conversion to glucose in our bodies. Glucose raises blood sugar, which in turn causes an increase in insulin levels. It's a no-brainer to understand that this is especially important to diabetics, but how does it affect non-diabetics?

Our bodies perform best when blood sugar level is kept relatively constant. If blood sugar drops too low, you feel lethargic, and/or hungry. It makes me plain ol' grumpy. When blood sugar takes a sudden rise, your body produces more insulin. Insulin brings the blood sugar level back down, primarily by converting the excess sugar to stored fat. (Say what?)

In my research, I found this link,

http://nutritiondata.self.com/topics/glycemic-index#ixzz20FINKjyk

The more quickly you increase your blood sugar, the more likely your body is to release an excess amount of insulin, and drive your blood sugar back down too low. Therefore, when you eat foods that cause a large and rapid glycemic response, you may feel an initial elevation in energy and mood as your blood sugar rises, but this is followed by a cycle of increased fat storage, lethargy, and more hunger! Roller coasters may be fun, but this one is not.

Should you remove all high-glucose foods from your diet? For non-diabetics, there are times when an increase in blood sugar and the rapid increase in insulin it causes may be just what the coach ordered. For example, after strenuous physical activity, insulin also helps move glucose into muscle cells, where it aids tissue repair. Because of this, some coaches and physical trainers recommend high-glycemic-index foods (such as sports drinks) immediately after exercise to speed recovery.

Also, the article said it's not Glycemic Index alone that leads to the increase in blood sugar. Equally important is the *amount* of the food that you consume. That's what *I'm* talkin' about! I love it when research backs up my message.

What does the Bible have to say about this?

All man's efforts are for his mouth, yet his appetite is never satisfied.
Ecc. 6:7

While losing weight, did I consider "glycemic index" when deciding what to eat? No, but I will now, but only in a vague, how much sugar, starch and carbs kind of way. Will I remove glucose/AKA sugar from my diet? No. Will I be vigilant of how much sugar I consume? You bet your buns I will. "Knowledge is power," is not just a cliché, it's the truth.

Chapter Thirteen
Obesity Connection to Cancer, Diabetes and Other Diseases
A Cautionary Chapter

Don't expect a lot of humor in this chapter. There is nothing funny about the diseases caused by obesity. Do expect warning, preaching, begging, nagging, and some strong encouragement to get healthy by attaining, and maintaining a healthy weight.

I am amazed, and alarmed by the vast number of health problems caused from being overweight. One that surprised even me was the connection between obesity and bone health. Logic would suggest that carrying around extra pounds would make your bones stronger – not so according a study at the University of Georgia which revealed that people who had a higher level of body fat had bones that were considerably weaker than those with lower levels of body fat.

Here is what Richard D. Lewis, a professor of foods and nutrition at the UGA College of Family and Consumer Sciences had to say about it. "Obesity is an epidemic in this country, and I think this study is critical because it highlights another potential negative health effect that people haven't considered,"

Carrying around extra pounds also increases wear and tear on weight bearing joints, such as knees, hips and spine. Is that slice of cheese cake worth the pain?

It is commonly accepted that obesity puts you at a higher risk for Type II diabetes. Here is my non-medical interpretation of what happens: while you continue to eat more than your body needs for fuel, you cause your pancreas to produce more and more insulin, until it becomes ineffectual. Your body is yelling "Wolf!" er I mean "Sugar!" And eventually the pancreas gives up on saving you. (I told you it was non-medical)

So what about cancer? Did you know that extra fat in your body actually increases the concentration of estrogen – a known cause of breast cancer? Estrogen levels also affect ovarian cancer and/or the treatment.

Clinical depression is often linked to obesity. Of course most people feel guilt, shame, anger, and a number of other emotions when they are overweight. We can't blame it all on America's obsession with being skinny. I suggest that poor nutrition causes a chemical imbalance in our brains. In the previous chapter I talked about sugar and starches in the diet and how they affect weight gain or loss. If you have ever known, lived with, or worked with someone suffering from diabetes, or hypoglycemia you know how their blood sugar levels influence their mood, disposition, and especially their reasoning powers. Even for a person with no severe health problems, sweets give you a high, followed by a noticeable low. Compare it to a drinking binge – fun and games, right? The low is the equivalent of a hangover.

God has equipped most of us with common sense about what and how much to eat. Consider this Biblical warning.

Do not join those who drink too much wine or gorge themselves on meat,

for drunkards and gluttons become poor, and drowsiness clothes them in rags. Proverbs 23:20-21 (NIV)

Chapter Fourteen
Coping with Stress

We encounter stressful situations every day. Some are more difficult than others. While writing this book, I found myself in yet another stressful situation.

I would like to tell you that I worked through the challenging time without reverting to my old habit of turning to food for comfort. Unfortunately, I didn't. The scales fluctuated in direct opposition to my mood. When I was down, the scales went up, and vice-versa. At the beginning of the book I said that I don't have deep-seated emotional problems, but that I simply love food. That being said, I admit to seeking comfort from food in trying times.

Worse than the stress-eating, the social eating really did me in, mostly at pot-luck-type events. And it wasn't because I didn't want to hurt someone's feelings by not tasting their food. I *did* taste, and it was *good*. So I ate *more*. I prepared special dishes, and I tasted them, too. You have to do that, right?

I'd been coasting on the maintenance train for too long. I got off at the junction of Ooh That Looks Good, and I'll Just Have a Little More, but missed the train when it left the station. (insert cartoon of railroad handcar) Eventually I gained back ten pounds. I fought hard against my food addiction. I'd lose two pounds, and then gain one, or both, back the next day.

Then one morning my spiritual alarm clock went off at 3:00 A. M. I tried to ignore it, but forty-five minutes later I gave in and got up. On the bookshelf beside my bed was a book I had received as a gift, "The Source of My Strength," by Charles Stanley. I'd never opened it.

Really, God? I know where my strength comes from. I think I may have actually rolled my eyes.

Being the obedient, practical, cock-eyed-optimistic person I am, I dusted off the book and thumbed through it. Here is what I found; or rather what found me.

My grace is sufficient for you, for My strength is made perfect in weakness.
2 Cor. 12:9

Yes, I'd read that Bible verse many times, but I needed to be reminded. I was trying to do it all in my own strength, and I have no strength. But I have faith, and I know where to turn for comfort and/or guidance. No, I'm not talking about Facebook, Twitter, or The Donut Shack. The first place we should turn to for help is often the last place we go. At that point I would have been on my face in prayer, but the carpet needed vacuuming, and my donut would have gotten dust bunnies all over it. Oops, I said that out loud, didn't I?

Lest I get bogged down in should-have, could-have, would-haves, I *had* to go back to what I know works: count and limit calories consumed, and get moving. Writing about it was hard. Doing it *again*, was even harder.

Everyone has a life-story. In order for me to write a story, I need to like the main character The writer spends a lot of time with that character.

Problem was, I was the main character in this story, and I didn't like me. To paraphrase Pogo, "I have met the enemy, and he is me."

In a good story, the main character must suffer. Carrying around additional weight makes my joints hurt – suffering. Check. The main character – that would be me -- must face hardships. Allowing myself to feel hunger – hardship, both physical and emotional. Check. I must overcome obstacles. A day that I don't overeat – overcoming weight battle. Check (every day I succeed).

I have participated in weight loss programs that claim you don't ever have to feel hunger. Those never worked for me. Not only must I accept an occasional feeling of true, stomach rumbling hunger, but know that because of it, I'm making real progress.

All hard work brings a profit, but mere talk leads only to poverty.
Proverbs 14: 23 (NIV)

It was time to stop talking about it, and do the hard work. I was weighed down, not only with fat, but with guilt, too. Here I was writing a book about weight loss, for goodness sake, and I couldn't even follow my own advice.

One day I went with my husband to a church luncheon. I was feeling especially fat and U-G-L-Y. Of course there was good food, and it was plentiful!

While I stood outside waiting for my husband, a friend walked by and said, "You have really lost the weight." I smiled and said, "Thank you," when I really wanted to scream, "Are you crazy? Can't you see how fat I am?"

As if that weren't enough; while sitting at the table visiting after the meal, a woman I barely know looked at me and said, "You know, you are beautiful."

"Who, me?" I squeaked. I certainly didn't *feel* beautiful. I felt old, fat, and ugly. She probably needed to see her optometrist. Bless her heart.

The bottom line is that it doesn't matter what someone else says or thinks about you. What matters is what you think or say to yourself – but more important is what God's word says about you and to you.

I praise you because I am fearfully and wonderfully made:
Your works are wonderful. I know that full well. Ps 139:14
(NIV)

In the same sense, it's not all about us. Our purpose as Christians is to bring glory to God. How can we do that if we are abusing His creation, or ignoring the sacrifice Jesus made for us?

> *Therefore, I urge you, brothers, in view of God's mercy, to offer*
> *your bodies as living sacrifices, holy and pleasing to God –*
> *this is your spiritual act of worship.*
> *Romans 12:1 (NIV)*

We cannot do that by starving ourselves, or by stuffing ourselves in the sinful act of gluttony.

Almost any addiction is destructive, and I had only gotten my addiction temporarily under control, and was on the verge totally of losing control. And somehow I had to take charge of my eating habits again. Fortunately I came to my senses before I went completely off the deep end. My health was more important than my love of food. I needed help! So I turned to the Bible for more words of wisdom.

> *"No temptation has seized you except what is common to man.*
> *and God is faithful," he will not let you be tempted beyond*
> *what you can bear. But when you are tempted, he will also*
> *provide a way out so that you can stand up under it.*
> *I Cor. 10:13 (NIV)*

Another problem: I don't always recognize God's help when it comes. I'm like the woman caught in a flood. She made it to the roof of her house and prayed, "God save me!" She truly believed that God would miraculously save her. Soon some neighbors came by in a fishing boat. They called out to her to get in the boat. The woman refused their help, stating, "God will save me."

Reluctantly, the neighbors left her there. The waters rose higher. Local firefighters arrived in an inflatable life raft and beckoned the woman to get into the raft. Again she refused, saying, "God will save me."

The waters rose even higher and the woman had to crawl to the very peak of the roof. A rescue team in a helicopter arrived and hovered overhead. The woman waved them off, saying, "God will save me." Just then the house collapsed. The woman was swept away in the swirling waters and drowned.

When she got to heaven, she complained bitterly to St. Peter. "Why didn't God save me?"

St. Peter scratched his head. "What are you talking about woman? God sent you a fishing boat, a life raft, and a helicopter!"

When you pray for help, be sure you are not *missing the boat* when it arrives, even if it's not the kind you expect. The waters are rising.

Chapter Fifteen
Train up a Child

Does anybody do that now? Yes, we do, whether we plan to or not. We train not only by our words, but by actions, which have even more impact. Children are little sponges, and it doesn't matter what is there for the soaking up; good, bad, or indifferent.

We were sponges, too. At some point we became saturated, and some of the "stuff" has started to *leak out*. Don't believe me? Have your mother's words ever spilled from your mouth?

Anita Renfroe has written and performs "The Mom Song," a hilarious version of all the things we say to our children on an average day. We've all said them, but think about what you're saying with your deeds.

We say, "You need to eat a good breakfast," while tossing back a latte and wolfing down a honey bun on the way to carpool. Wipe mouth. "It's the most important meal of the day." Sponges absorb – good breakfast = high caffeine and high carbs/sugar.

But in defense of moms everywhere, we're busy. We don't have time to cook breakfast, and our picky children probably wouldn't eat it if we did. Besides, breakfast is served at school, so no problem. Right?

I checked local school breakfast menus and found that they offer a reasonably healthy fare, but it still comes down to choices. Will your children choose to eat it? There is an unhealthy addiction in our country and it didn't just begin. Count the number of senior citizens in the McDonalds' dining room. How would I know this? I'm from the generation that first discovered the joys of fast food. Forget the pot of gold at the end of the rainbow; there's a supersized order of golden fries waiting for you under those glowing arches.

Just as I can't blame church fellowships for gluttony, neither can I blame McDonalds or any other fast-food chain for our bad habits. These businesses have merely responded to the market demands. The tide does seems to be turning, be it every so slow. Many restaurants are posting caloric and nutritional values. The choices are ours. They always have been.

How do we undo habits learned from three generations of poor choices? We train by example. Make coffee at home. It's not that hard, and you will save money. There are some nice travel mugs that keep it hot, but make certain it has a good-fitting lid. I don't want you to sue me if you were to spill hot liquid on a sensitive part of your body.

My next suggestion requires some planning on your part. Get up early enough to make your breakfast at home, too. There are some healthy choices that are quick and easy to prepare. And *do not* eat in the car. It's messy and potentially dangerous. Did you know more accidents are caused by people eating while driving than while talking on their cell phones?

That takes care of breakfast, but what about the other meals. Again, this takes planning. Take your lunch to work; anything from a sandwich to a three-course meal. I've mentioned the health advantages to whole-grain products. Make your sandwich with high fiber, whole grain bread, and lean meat, or even vegetables. A southern favorite is a tomato sandwich, "mater samich" in the vernacular. (Word of advice, don't put the parts together until you are ready to eat – can we say soggy.) Also, light mayonnaise has a much improved taste these days.

If you want a more hearty meal, dish up some leftovers from a meal you prepared. There are handy containers made especially for that purpose. You can even freeze meals in them. Most work places have microwaves in employee break rooms.

There are also some good choices available in the frozen section of your grocery store. Read the labels for calories, carbs, and sodium content. Since they are often loaded with sodium, I don't recommend a constant diet of these, but they are better for you than a burger and fries.

Sometimes when I meet with my writers' group for a "writing marathon" we bring a potluck meal. My writer friends are health conscious, good cooks.

By all means, **<u>Stay Away from the Vending Machines</u>**! Something wicked this way comes. Trust me.

The Hunger Games

What and how much we eat is one of the few things we are in total control of – until it controls us. The Bible has much to say about hunger, both physical and spiritual hunger, and how we are to approach it. It also has instruction as to how we are to respond to the hunger of others.

Ps 107:9 *… for he satisfies the thirsty and fills the hungry with good things.*

Ps 146:7 *He upholds the cause of the oppressed and gives food to the hungry.*

The Lord sets prisoners free.

Mt 5:6 *Blessed are those who hunger and thirst for*
 righteousness.

Lk 1:53 *He has filled the hungry with good things but has sent the rich away empty*

Lk 6:21 *Blesssed are you who hunger now, for you will be satisfied. Blessed are you who weep now, for you will laugh.*

Jn 6:5 *When Jesus looked up and saw a great multitude coming toward him,*
 he said to Phillip, "Where shall we buy bread for these people to eat.?

6. He asked this only to test him, for he already had in mind what he was going

to do.

Php 4:12 *I know what it is to be in need, and I know what it is to have plenty.*

I have learned to be content in every situation, whether well-fed or hungry,

whether living in plenty or want.

13. I can do everything through him who gives me strength.

I've only chosen a few. There are many more. I'm not saying that you can pray your way to thin. But I am saying that confessing the sin of gluttony, and turning it over to the Lord will help you to realize what you are doing to your body, God's temple, and convict you to turn to healthy eating practices. Overeating, or gluttony, leads to obesity. Obesity leads to death, either slowly or quickly.

Does your desire for food control you, or do you control your appetite?

A few paragraphs above, I stated that the Bible also has much to say about what we are to do about the hunger of others. (insert mental picture of starving children with haunted eyes and bloated stomachs) America is, as a whole, a well-fed, but generous nation. Even people living in poverty in the United States have options for feeding themselves and their children. Government assistance programs, religious and humanitarian organizations are available if we chose to accept their help.

I am not here to criticize these programs. On the contrary, I applaud them and am happy to support to them with tax dollars and private donations.

In the last few years our family income has shrunk, and our expenses have grown. Sadly, we've had to reduce or even eliminate some of our contributions. In light of this I have to consider how I would feel if we were truly hungry and in need. Would I share what meager resources I have, or would I hoard every crumb?

Imagine if the United States were to suffer, God forbid, a catastrophic economic collapse. (This is not the prelude to a political statement.) There are many factors that could precipitate such an event. In the Old Testament something like this is referred to as "a famine." Such an event can be brought on by pestilence, drought, earthquakes, floods, changing weather patterns that disrupt growing seasons, war, and countless other scenarios.

My parents and my husband's parents lived through "The Great Depression." They taught us a lot about surviving on little, but at the same time raised us in a time of plenty. I realize that sounds contradictory, but we listened to their stories of endurance and ingenuity. One of my mother's favorite sayings was "Waste not, want not."

As a child, did I waste? Oh yeah.

Did I want? Not for much.

Sample Food Diary

Date:　/　/　/　　　　Time and Food eaten　　　　Calories

Breakfast:
Protein　　_____　　　_____
Dairy　　　_____　　　_____
Fruit　　　_____　　　_____
....

Mid-morning snack:
Dairy or Protein_____　　　_____
....

Lunch:
Protein　　_____　　　_____
Dairy　　　_____　　　_____
Fruit　　　_____　　　_____
....

Afternoon Snack:
Dairy or Protein_____　　　_____
....

Dinner:
Entrée　　　_____　　　_____
Vegetable　_____　　　_____
Fruit　　　_____　　　_____
Dessert　　_____　　　_____
....

Total glasses of Water: _____　　　Total calories: _____
Physical Activity: _____Time:_____ Calories burned:_____
Weight: _____

www.ingramcontent.com/pod-product-compliance
Lightning Source LLC
Chambersburg PA
CBHW071236280526
45787CB00002B/950